Asma Mensi

THE ROLE OF THE NURSE IN THE DIGESTIVE ENDOSCOPY ROOM

Asma Mensi

THE ROLE OF THE NURSE IN THE DIGESTIVE ENDOSCOPY ROOM

ScienciaScripts

Imprint

Any brand names and product names mentioned in this book are subject to trademark, brand or patent protection and are trademarks or registered trademarks of their respective holders. The use of brand names, product names, common names, trade names, product descriptions etc. even without a particular marking in this work is in no way to be construed to mean that such names may be regarded as unrestricted in respect of trademark and brand protection legislation and could thus be used by anyone.

Cover image: www.ingimage.com

This book is a translation from the original published under ISBN 978-620-6-70655-7.

Publisher:
Sciencia Scripts
is a trademark of
Dodo Books Indian Ocean Ltd. and OmniScriptum S.R.L publishing group

120 High Road, East Finchley, London, N2 9ED, United Kingdom
Str. Armeneasca 28/1, office 1, Chisinau MD-2012, Republic of Moldova, Europe
Printed at: see last page
ISBN: 978-620-7-77148-6

CONTENTS

INTRODUCTION

Endoscopy, also known as digestive fibroscopy, is a medical imaging examination designed to visualize and explore the inner lining of the digestive tract through a flexible cable inserted through the mouth or anus, and equipped with a lighting system and a miniaturized video camera. This examination, performed for diagnostic or therapeutic purposes, generally requires a light general anaesthetic and a short hospital stay. There are two types of digestive endoscopy: upper and lower (or colonoscopy) [1].

Upper gastrointestinal endoscopy enables us to observe the upper part of the digestive tract, i.e. the esophagus, stomach and duodenum. It is also known as gastroduodenal endoscopy or gastroduodenal fibroscopy. The examination is performed under local or general anaesthetic, using an endoscope. Sometimes, this instrument is used to take a sample, remove a tumor or foreign body, or coagulate blood vessels[2].

Gastrointestinal endoscopy, better known as colonoscopy, is an examination to observe or intervene inside the colon and rectum. This examination is prescribed by the attending physician when the patient complains of digestive symptoms such as diarrhea, persistent pain or the presence of blood in the stool. It may also be requested to detect or remove a cancerous or precancerous lesion. Over a million colonoscopies are performed in France every year[3].

Every endoscopic procedure, whether diagnostic or therapeutic, relies on a partnership between gastroenterologists and endoscopy nurses. The latter must be skilled in dexterity and mastery of the procedure, and able to anticipate the various stages of the examination. They must receive specific initial and ongoing training in order to master the various endoscopy techniques. [4]

Issues

Nurses are responsible for the quality and safety of the nursing care given to the patient in the run-up to digestive endoscopy, during and after the procedure, and in the disinfection and maintenance of medical equipment. They must have the necessary knowledge, training and experience to assist with digestive endoscopy.

They must be competent and capable of noticing any abnormality and notifying the doctor promptly. They must also know how to provide the necessary care to a patient facing possible complications, such as perforation, hemorrhage or choleperitoneum. The patient may experience diarrhea, hypotension or severe pain.

In view of these data, and given the importance of the nurse's role in the preparation and performance of digestive endoscopy. We have chosen to explore this subject in order to evaluate the role of the nurse in the digestive endoscopy room, and to identify the difficulties and problems that may be encountered when participating in the performance of this technique.

The research questions we need to ask are:

- Does the nurse have sufficient theoretical and practical knowledge of digestive endoscopy?
- Are there any difficulties that can influence the quality of nursing care provided during digestive endoscopy?
- What solutions can be envisaged to optimize the quality of nursing care provided during digestive endoscopy?

The general aim of our work is to evaluate the role of the nurse in the digestive endoscopy room and to identify any difficulties and obstacles that may influence the quality of nursing care provided during this procedure, and to put forward suggestions with a view to improving quality.

Our specific objectives are as follows:

- Evaluating the role of the nurse in the digestive endoscopy room ;
- Identify any difficulties and obstacles that may affect the quality of nursing care provided using this technique;
- Make suggestions to improve the quality of nursing care.

MATERIALS AND METHODS

1. TYPE OF STUDY

As part of our end-of-study project, we carried out a descriptive, quantitative, cross-sectional study of a sample of nurses working in digestive endoscopy units, with the aim of examining the role of the nurse in the digestive endoscopy room, identifying any difficulties and obstacles that may influence the quality of nursing care provided during this procedure, and proposing suggestions for quality improvement.

2. STUDY AREA

Our study was carried out in the endoscopy rooms of :

- Charles Nicolle University Hospital Gastrology Department
- Gastrology Department, Rabta University Hospital

3. DURATION OF STUDY

The study conducted in the above-mentioned departments lasted from February 12 to May 19, 2023.

4. THE TARGET POPULATION OF OUR STUDY

At the outset, we wanted our study to reach as many nurses as possible, with a minimum of 40, but given the time constraints and availability of nurses, we were only able to distribute 20 questionnaires.

5. INCLUSION CRITERIA

Our population includes all nurses who work on the days of our visits to the above-mentioned gastrology departments, regardless of rank, gender or seniority.

6. NON-INCLUSION CRITERIA

Senior technicians, orderlies and student trainees are not included in our population.

7. DATA COLLECTION TOOL

Information was collected by means of a self-administered questionnaire to the nurses who agreed to take part in our study. Our questionnaire was written in French and consisted of 26 questions.

- 5 questions relating to the identification of nurses ;
- 7 questions on theoretical knowledge of digestive endoscopy;
- 10 about practical knowledge
- 2. Questions about difficulties encountered.
- 2 questions about continuing education.

8. THE INQUIRY

As part of a pre-survey, we observed and interviewed 4 nurses working in the gastrology department of Charles Nicolle University Hospital, to find out if there were any gaps or poorly-written questions.

9. DATA PROCESSING TOOLS

We used Microsoft Office Excel 2019 to interpret and analyze the information gathered.

Graphical and tabular representations were made using the same Microsoft Office Excel software.

10. ETHICAL CONSIDERATIONS

We began by seeking the agreement and consent of the nurses working in the selected departments.

Similarly, we have explained to all the nurses who agreed to take part in our survey that the information will be treated in complete confidentiality and with respect for their anonymity.

11. THE DIFFICULTIES ENCOUNTERED

We encountered no difficulties except for the refusal of some nurses to take part in our survey, and a lack of time which prevented us from reaching the desired number of nurses.

RESULTS

IDENTIFYING THE TARGET POPULATION

1.   Genre :

Two-thirds of our population (67%) are women, with a sex ratio of 0.49.

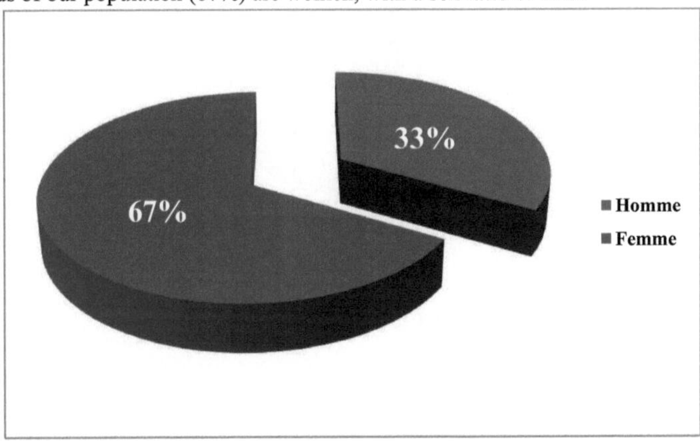

Chart 1: Breakdown by gender

2.   Age :

A third of our population (33%) are aged between 41 and 50.

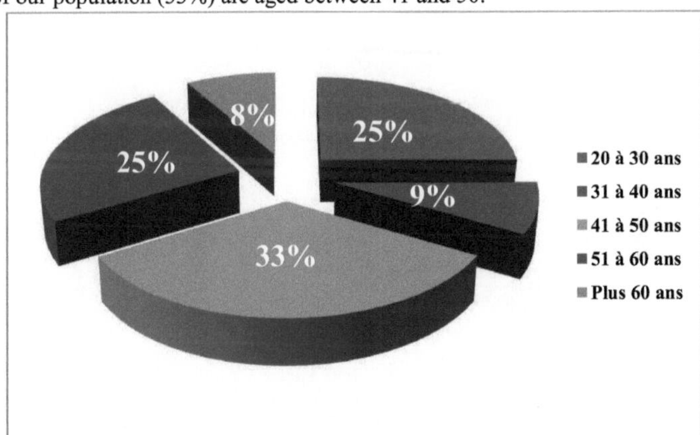

Chart 2: Age distribution

3.   Grade

Half of our population (50%) are nursing majors.

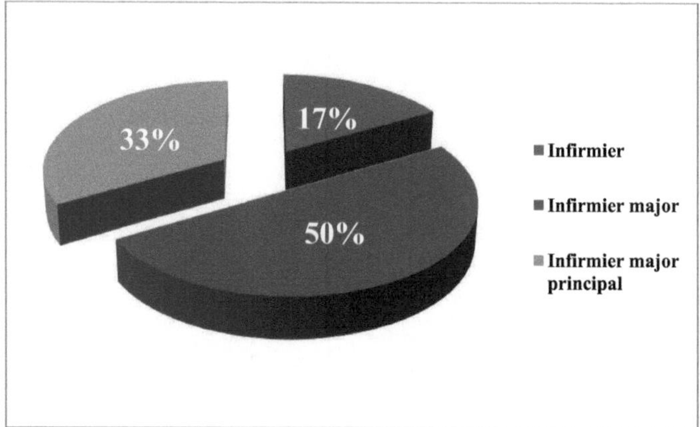

Figure 3: Breakdown by grade

4.   Seniority in the nursing profession

Three-quarters of our population (75%) have been with us for more than 5 years

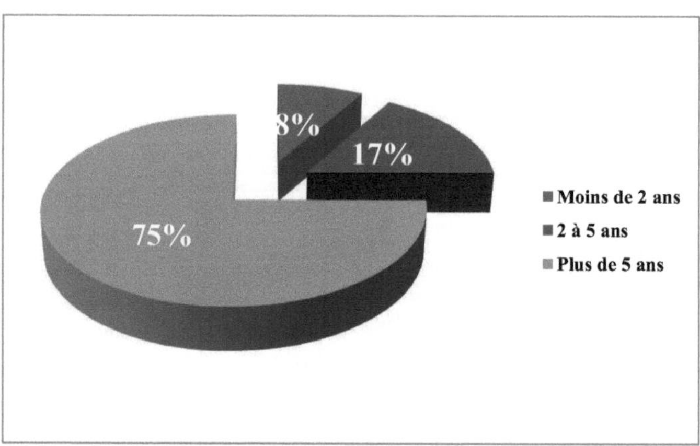

Figure 4: Breakdown by seniority in the nursing profession

5.   Length of service in current department

Forty-two percent of our population have been with their current company for more than 5 years.

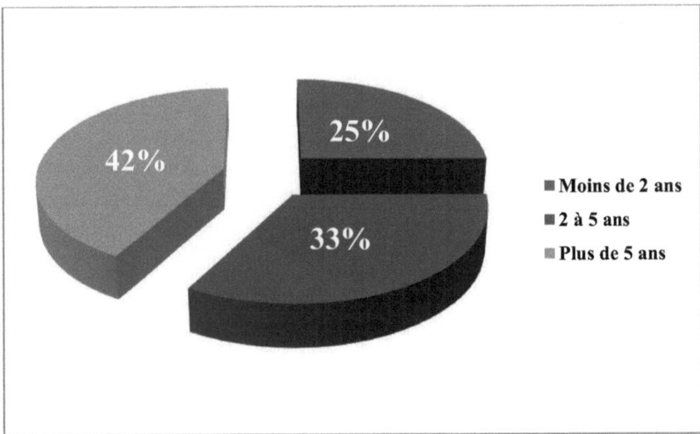

Figure 5: Breakdown by length of service in current department

THEORETICAL KNOWLEDGE

6.   Specific training in digestive endoscopy

Two-thirds of our population indicate that they have received specific training in digestive endoscopy .

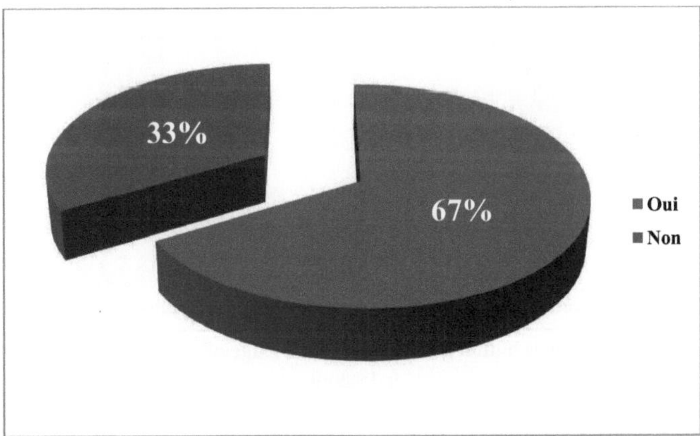

Chart 6: Breakdown by specific training in digestive endoscopy

7. Type of training received

Sixty-two percent of our population indicate that their training in digestive endoscopy comes from basic education (basic training).

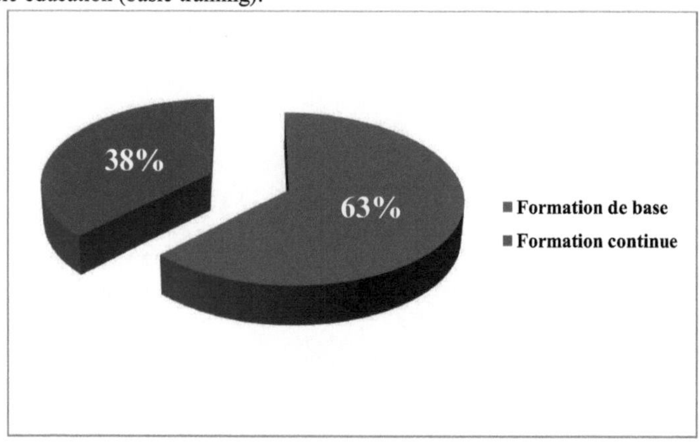

Figure 7: Breakdown by type of training received

8. Definition of digestive endoscopy

40% of nurses surveyed gave wrong answers regarding the definition of endoscopy

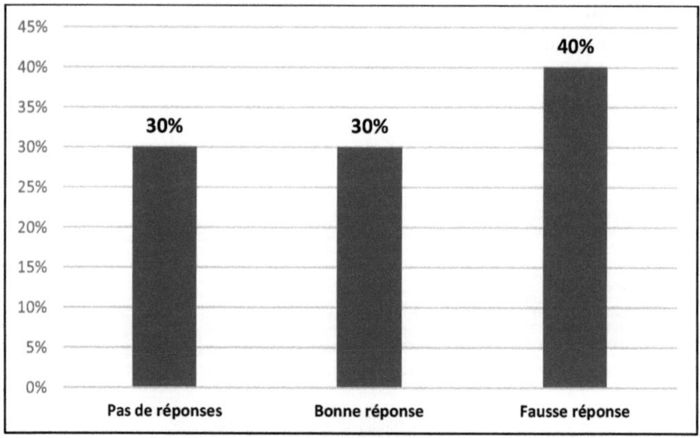

Chart 8: Distribution according to knowledge of the definition of endoscopy

9.   The different types of digestive endoscopy

A majority of 98% cited fibroscopy

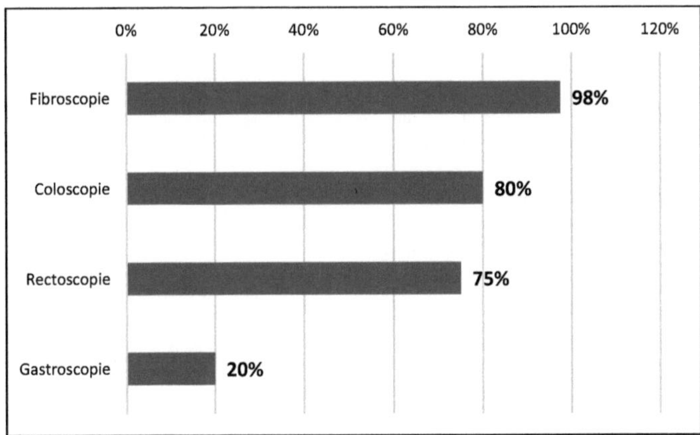

Figure 9: Distribution according to knowledge of the different types of **digestive** endoscopy

10.   The main indications for upper GI endoscopy

Among the main indications for upper GI endoscopy, 92% of our population cited the diagnosis and follow-up of GI haemorrhage, and the diagnosis and follow-up of peptic ulcers.

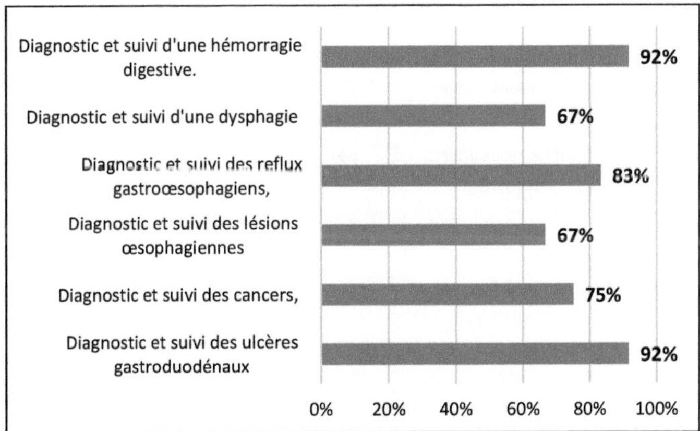

Figure 10: Distribution according to knowledge of the main indications for **upper** GI endoscopy

11. Main indications for lower GI endoscopy

Among the indications for lower GI endoscopy, 83% mentioned screening for colonic tumor risk factors.

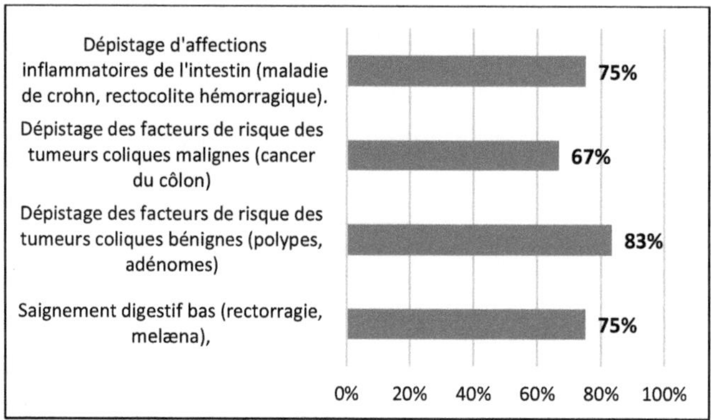

Figure 11: Breakdown by main indications for lower GI endoscopy

12. The main risks of digestive endoscopy

Among the main risks that can arise during digestive endoscopy, 75% cited perforation of the digestive wall.

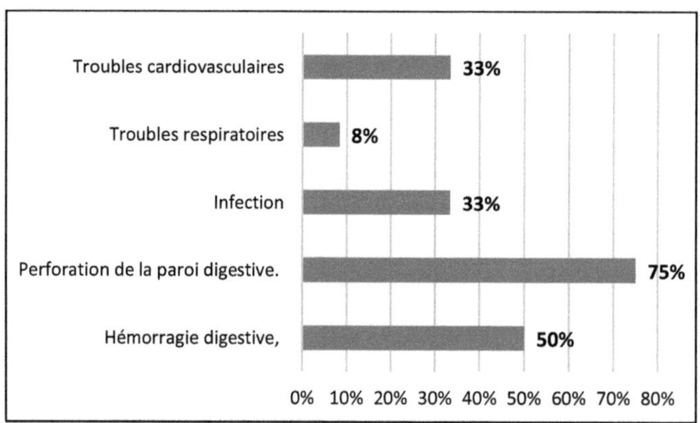

Figure 12: Distribution according to knowledge of the main risks that can arise during **digestive** endoscopy

13.   Activities in the digestive endoscopy room

The activities to be carried out in the digestive endoscopy room are shown in the chart below.

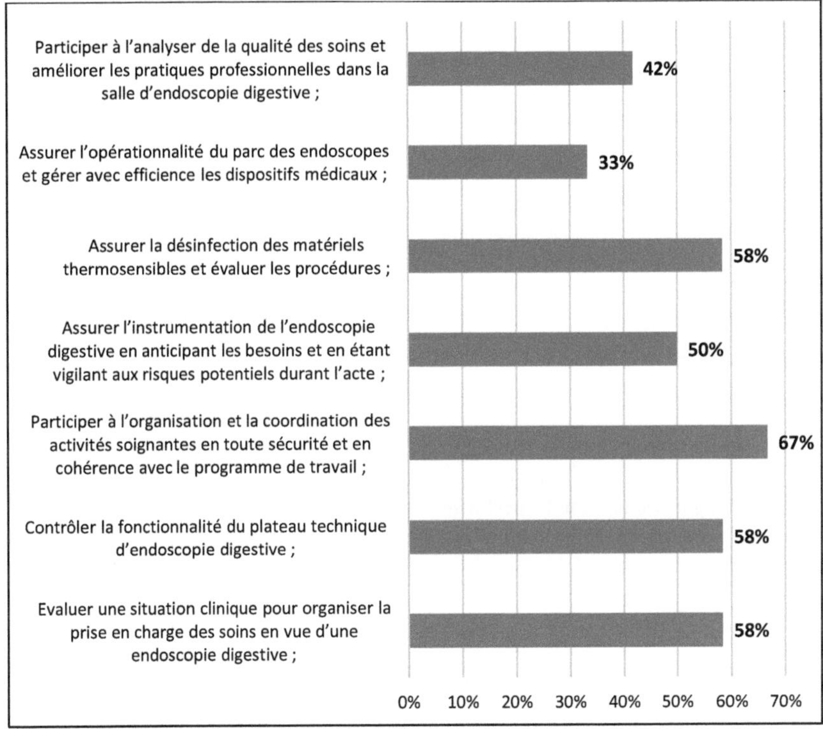

Chart 13: Breakdown by activities to be performed in the digestive endoscopy room

14. Nursing procedures to be performed prior to digestive endoscopy

The steps to be taken before performing a digestive endoscopy are listed in the chart below.

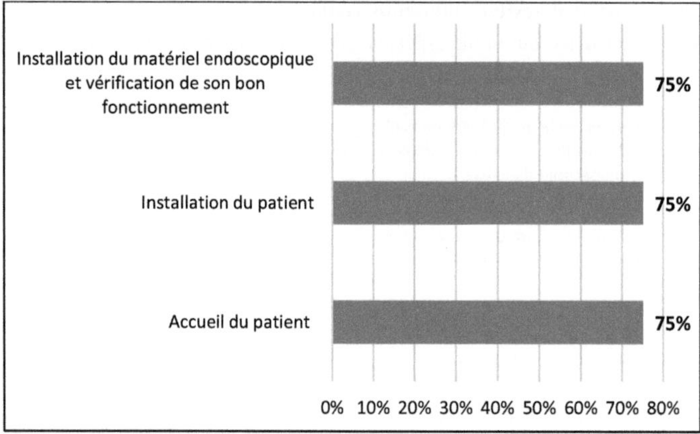

Chart 14: Breakdown of nursing procedures performed prior to digestive endoscopy

15. Nursing procedures to be performed during digestive endoscopy

The nursing procedures to be carried out during digestive endoscopy are shown in the following chart.

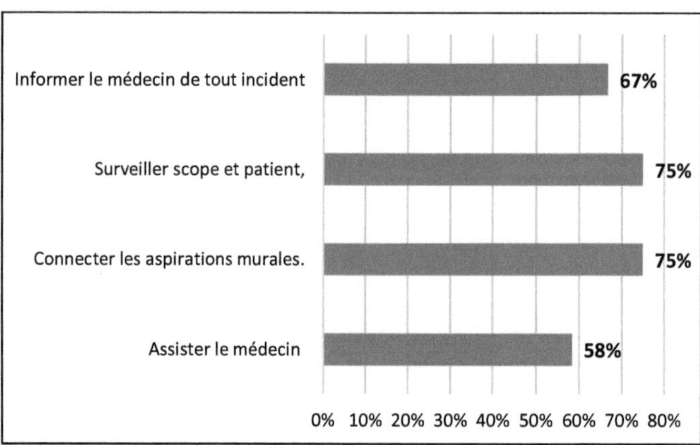

Chart 15: Breakdown of nursing procedures performed during **digestive** endoscopy

16. What nursing procedures do you perform after a digestive endoscopy?

The nursing procedures to be performed after a digestive endoscopy are shown in the following chart:

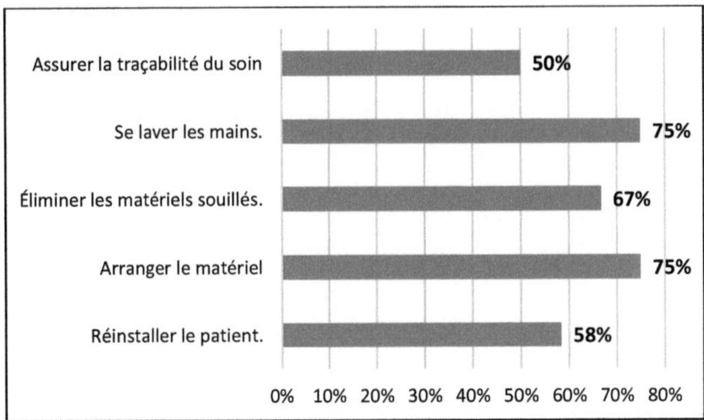

Chart 16: Distribution according to the Nursing procedures to be performed after digestive endoscopy

17. General hygiene precautions to be observed when participating in digestive endoscopy?

The general hygiene precautions to be observed when participating in digestive endoscopy are illustrated in the following chart.

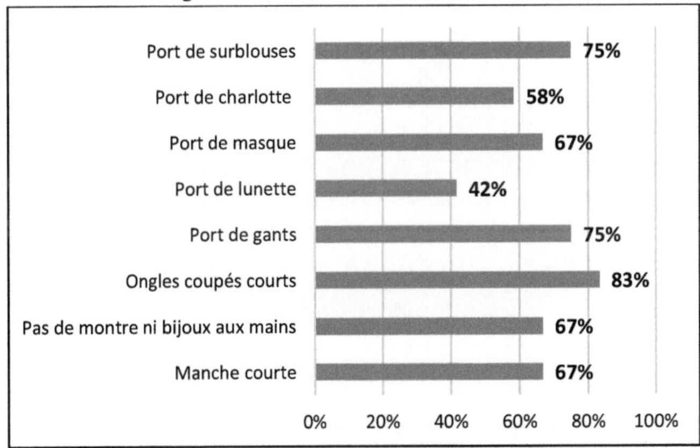

Figure 17: Distribution according to general hygiene precautions to be observed when participating in digestive endoscopy

18.   Endoscope disinfection in the digestive endoscopy room
A majority of 83% of nurses say they disinfect endoscopes in the endoscopy room.

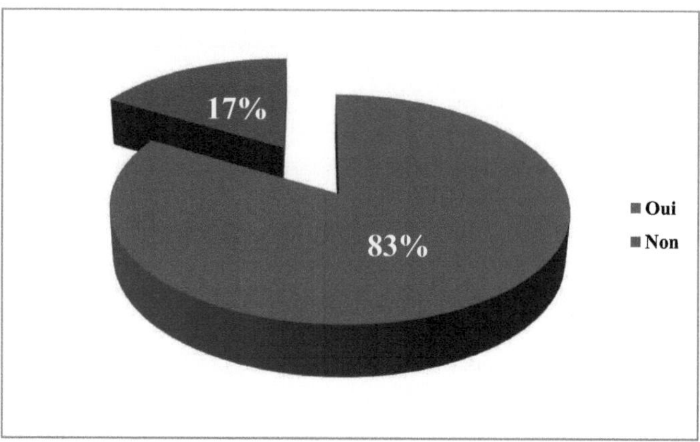

Figure 18: Breakdown of endoscope disinfection in the **digestive**
endoscopy room, by type of disinfection performed

19.   Are you familiar with endoscope cleaning and disinfection procedures?
95% of nurses say they are familiar with endoscope cleaning and disinfection procedures

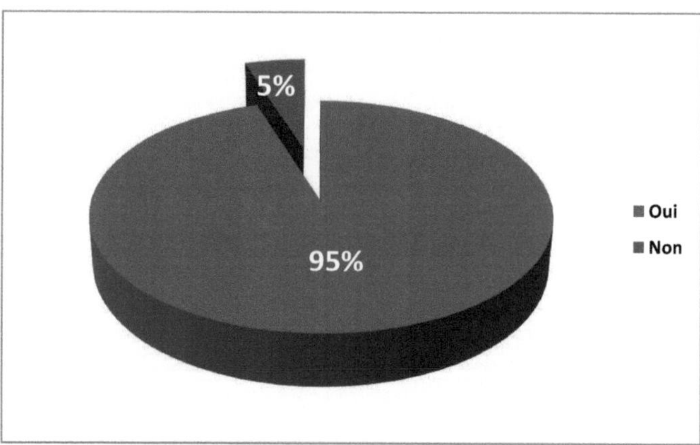

Figure 19: Distribution according to knowledge of endoscope cleaning and
disinfection procedures

20. Endoscope cleaning and disinfection procedures

Only 20% of nurses test the endoscope for leaks before cleaning, and check the endoscope before storage.

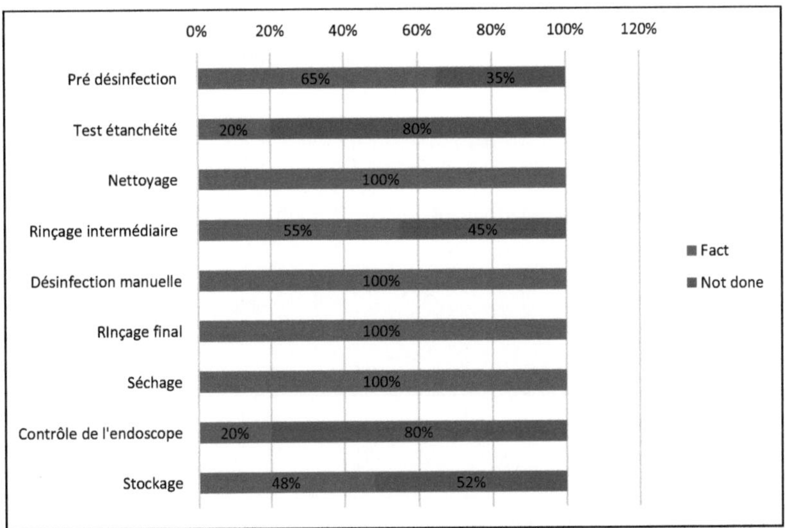

Figure 20: Breakdown by endoscope cleaning and disinfection procedure

21. Difficulties influencing the quality of nursing care during digestive endoscopy

A majority of 83% of nurses indicate that they have encountered difficulties that influence the quality of nursing care provided during a digestive endoscopy.

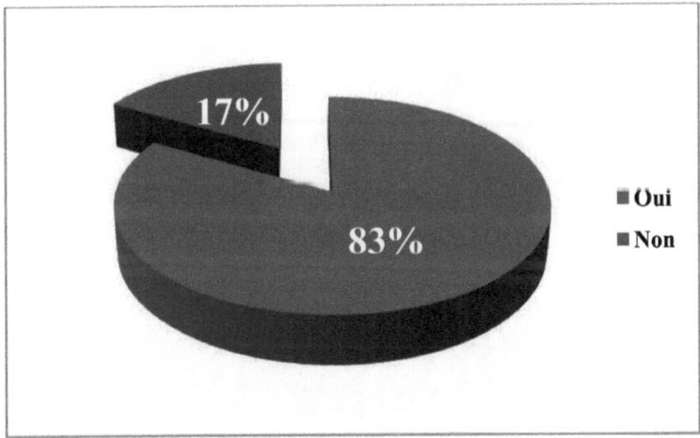

Figure 21: Distribution according to difficulties influencing the quality of nursing care provided during **digestive** endoscopy

22.   Type of difficulties encountered

Staff shortages and work overload are the difficulties most mentioned by 90% of our nurses.

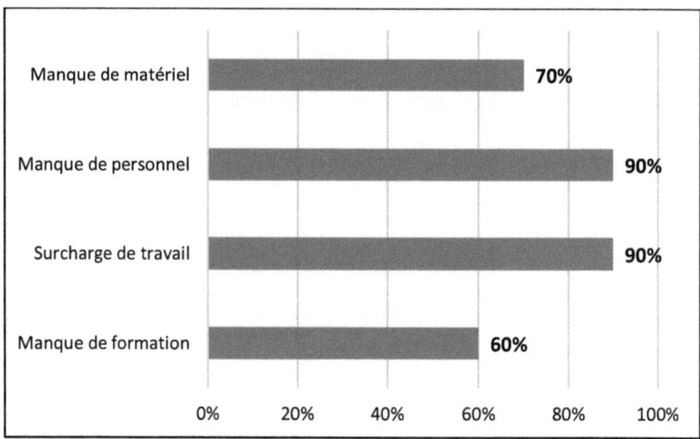

Figure 22: Breakdown by type of difficulty encountered

ONGOING TRAINING NEEDS

23.   Need for additional training in digestive endoscopy

Three-quarters of our nurses (75%) say they need further training in digestive endoscopy.

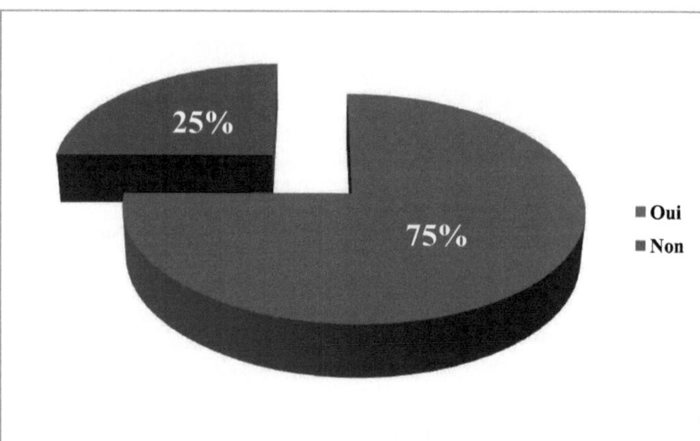

Figure 23: Breakdown by need for additional training in digestive
endoscopy

24.   the topics on which you would like to be trained?

Slightly less than half of the nurses surveyed would like to participate in continuing education sessions on equipment cleaning and disinfection procedures.

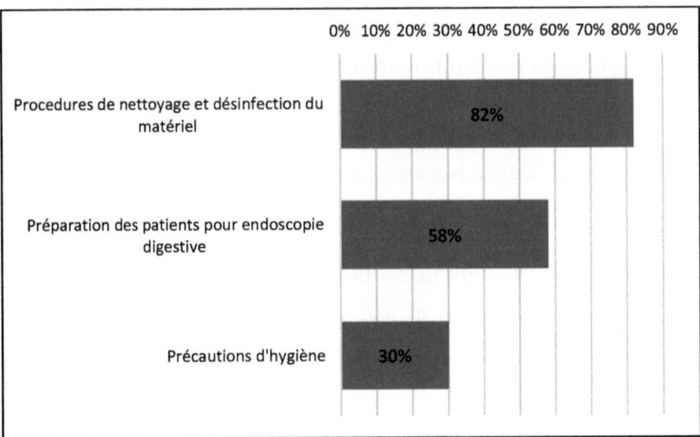

Figure 24: Breakdown by need for additional training in digestive endoscopy

DISCUSSION

A study carried out to evaluate the role of the nurse in the digestive endoscopy room yielded the following data.

In terms of gender, our population is made up of 67% women and 33% men, with a sex ratio of 4.9.

About age 25% of our population are aged between 20 and 30, while 8% are aged between 31 and 40, 33% are aged between 41 and 50, however 25% are aged between 51 and 60 and 8% are aged over 60 with an average age of 43.3.

In terms of grade, our population is made up of 17% nurses, 50% major nurses and 33% principal major nurses.   .

About seniority in the nursing profession 8% have been nurses for less than 2 years, 17% for 2 to 5 years and 75% for more than 5 years.

Regarding seniority in the current department, our population is made up of 25% of nurses with a seniority of less than 2 years, while 33% have a seniority of 2 to 5 years and 42% have a seniority of more than 5 years.

Regarding training, 67% of our population indicate that they have received specific training in digestive endoscopy. Of these, 63% indicate that they have received basic training (Enseignement de base).

Although 30% of the nurses gave no answers concerning the definition of endoscopy, only 30% gave a correct definition and 30% gave wrong answers.

These data clearly show a lack of knowledge among nurses, many of whom are unaware of the definition of endoscopy, which is a well-known and widespread diagnostic and therapeutic procedure. Indeed, endoscopy is a generic term meaning "to look inside". This technology has been in development for over 150 years, with the first rigid endoscopes dating back to 1852. However, the real revolution came in the early 1970s, with the use of fiber optics and the appearance of the first flexible fiberscopes, which considerably enhanced technical performance and comfort compared with the old rigid devices.

Among the most pertinent definitions of digestive endoscopy is that found in VIDAL 2023, which states that digestive endoscopy, which may also be called digestive fibroscopy. It is a medical imaging examination designed to visualize and explore the inner wall of the digestive tract via a flexible cable inserted through the mouth or anus. This cable is equipped with a lighting system and a miniaturized video camera. This examination, performed for diagnostic or therapeutic purposes, generally requires a light general anaesthetic and a short hospital stay. There are two types of digestive endoscopy: upper and lower (or colonoscopy).

However, there are 2 types of endoscopes: fiberscopes and electronic endoscopes or videoendoscopes (axial and lateral vision).

Regarding the different types of endoscopy, several answers were given. Fibroscopy was mentioned by 98% of nurses, colonoscopy by 80%, rectoscopy by 75% and gastroscopy by 20%.

The main indications for upper GI endoscopy. Several indications have been mentioned. Diagnosis and follow-up of peptic ulcers, and diagnosis and follow-up of haemorrhage were mentioned by 92% of our nurses. The diagnosis and follow-up of gastroesophageal reflux disease was mentioned by 83%. However, the diagnosis and follow-up of cancer was mentioned by 75%, and the diagnosis and follow-up of esophageal lesions by 67%. Diagnosis and follow-up of dysphagia mentioned by 67%.

When asked about the main indications for lower GI endoscopy, 75% cited lower GI bleeding (rectal bleeding, melena), 83% cited screening for risk factors of benign colonic tumors (polyps, adenomas), 67% cited screening for risk factors of malignant colonic tumors (colon cancer), while 75% cited screening for inflammatory bowel disease (crohn's disease, ulcerative colitis).

Data collected from nurses working in endoscopy rooms reveal a lack of knowledge on the part of these caregivers. Indeed, various documents indicate that upper digestive endoscopy, which visualizes the esophagus, stomach and early small intestine; **[1.2.5]**

Whereas colonoscopy, or lower digestive endoscopy, visualizes the colon (large intestine) and rectum, as well as the terminal part of the small intestine. [**1.2.5**]

Upper endoscopy explores the upper digestive tract up to the 2nd or 3rd duodenum. It is a routine examination, performed as a first-line treatment for any symptom or condition requiring exploration of the upper digestive tract: dyspeptic disorders, abdominal pain, digestive bleeding (hematemesis or melena), dysphagia. However, there are several contraindications to upper endoscopy: digestive perforations, full stomachs: risk of inhalation pneumopathy, difficult or even dangerous introduction of the fiberscope in case of pharyngoesophageal diverticulum, decompensated cardiac or respiratory insufficiency, shock, consciousness disorders in a non-intubated patient[2.4.5].

There are several types of lower digestive endoscopy, such as anuscopies, which explore the anus, anal canal and lower rectum. Anoscopy is part of the proctological examination and requires no patient preparation. The main indications for anuscopies are rectal discharge, rectal syndrome, severe constipation, anal incontinence and anal pain. [5]

In addition to anoscopy, rectoscopy is used to visualize the rectum. Rectoscopy is indicated in cases of constipation, especially recent constipation, diarrhea that refuses to respond to standard treatment, rectal discharge, proctalgia, rectal syndrome, pelvic and left foscial pain, cachexia or severe anemia, and bloody or non-bloody discharge outside the defecation.

Colonoscopy is designed to visualize the colon. It is indicated for screening polyps and cancers in at-risk subjects, with a history of inflammatory bowel disease, a family history of familial polyposis, a family history of polyps or colonic cancer (from the age of 45) and any persistent colonic symptoms, especially after the age of 50, as well as intestinal transit disorders: diarrhoea, constipation, alternating diarrhoea and constipation [5].
Colonoscopy is also indicated for abdominal pain, chronic diarrhoea and rectal discharge, even if associated with haemorrhoidal pathology, and for the assessment of iron-deficiency anaemia[5].
As for the main risks that can arise during digestive endoscopy, several were mentioned. Digestive hemorrhage was mentioned by 50% of nurses, perforation of the digestive wall by 75%, infection by 33%, respiratory problems by 8% and cardiovascular problems by 33%.

Although an acceptable number of nursing staff cited a few risks attributed to endoscopy, a great deal of unfamiliarity was noted among many of them regarding the risks to which patients are exposed during endoscopy. Indeed, various documents mention that there are different risks that can be generated by endoscopy. These risks can be divided into three main categories: infectious risks, threats to staff safety and environmental risks[6].

Infectious risks may come from an exogenous source, i.e. the patient's immediate environment (e.g. use of multipurpose endoscopy rooms for bronchoscopies and colonoscopies without negative pressure, and the number of air changes required recovery rooms used by unknowingly colonized clients)[6].

Infectious risks may arise from breakdowns in the reprocessing process or in the handling of endoscopes and accessories (failure of high-level disinfection or sterilization of endoscopes due to failure to comply with cleaning procedures, or contaminated endoscopes following wet storage) [6].

Infectious risks can also arise from an endogenous source related to the patient's clinical situation (state of health) and the type of procedure performed by the physician (e.g. endogenous flora and exogenous microbes)[6].

As far as personnel are concerned, infectious risks generally come from an exogenous source, either through contact with the immediate environment (from multi-purpose rooms used for bronchoscopies without negative pressure, the number of air changes required and activities related to reprocessing of endoscopes and accessories carried out in unsafe premises) or through contact with a sick patient, as well as airborne contamination (tuberculosis patient)[6].

Similarly, endoscopy can expose both caregiver and patient to an increased risk of exposure to blood and other biological fluids through pricks, cuts or splashes on the mucous membranes; the potential risk is linked to the presence of blood-borne viruses (HIV, HBV, HCV) due to failure to observe protective measures.[6] **The risk of exposure to blood and other biological** fluids through pricks, cuts or splashes on the mucous membranes is also increased.

Other risks to patients include physical injuries such as falls, lack of supervision and mobilization assistance, crowded conditions and accidental spills[6].

In terms of activities to be carried out by nurses in the digestive endoscopy room, 67% mentioned taking part in the organization and coordination of care activities, in complete safety and in line with the work schedule; 58% mentioned assessing a clinical situation to organize care management for digestive endoscopy, as well as monitoring the functionality of the digestive endoscopy technical platform and the disinfection of heat-sensitive equipment, and evaluating procedures. However, 50% mentioned the instrumentation of digestive endoscopy, anticipating needs and being vigilant to potential risks during the procedure; 40% mentioned participation in the analysis of the quality of care and the improvement of professional practices in the digestive endoscopy room; and 42% mentioned the operationality of the endoscope fleet and the efficient management of medical devices.

The roles of endoscopy nurses can be many and varied, but are generally common. In fact, they are involved in welcoming and informing patients, as well as preparing them physically and psychologically, all of which are areas where the endoscopy nurse's own role comes into play.

They have a duty to explain the examination and its risks, and to ensure that patients understand them. They are also responsible for patient comfort and safety, checking medical records and examination requests, blood tests, ensuring that colonic preparation has been carried out, that patients are fasting, and perfusing if necessary.

Regarding endoscope cleaning and disinfection procedures, 95% of nurses said they were familiar with them. However, although 100% mentioned cleaning, manual disinfection, final rinsing and drying, 65% mentioned pre-disinfection sla, 52% mentioned storage and only 20% mentioned endoscope leak testing, which must be carried out before cleaning, and endoscope inspection after disinfection and before storage.

When asked about the nursing procedures to be carried out prior to digestive endoscopy, 75% of nurses mentioned welcoming the patient, installing the patient and setting up the endoscopic equipment and checking that it is working properly.

As for the nursing acts to be carried out during digestive endoscopy, 75% cited the connection of wall aspirations and monitoring of the scope and patient, while 67% mentioned informing the doctor of any incident, and 58% assisting the doctor.

About nursing procedures to be performed after digestive endoscopy. Several actions were cited. These included arranging the equipment and washing hands, cited by 75% of nurses; disposing of dirty equipment, cited by 67%; reinstalling the patient, cited by 58%; arranging the equipment, cited by 75%; and tracing the care, cited by 50%.

These data clearly show that the essential role of the digestive endoscopy nurse is largely overlooked. Indeed, the tasks assigned to endoscopy nurses can be diverse and varied, but are generally common to many endoscopy centers.

Nurses play a very important role in digestive endoscopy rooms. In addition to instrumentation and the application of treatments, nurses have a very important role to play in welcoming patients, installing them, cleaning, disinfecting and storing endoscopes.

Welcoming the patient, providing information, and preparing him or her physically and psychologically, are all areas in which the endoscopy nurse plays a key role. They help to explain the examination and its risks, and check that the patient understands them. They ensure patient comfort and safety, check medical records and examination requests, blood tests, and make sure that colonic preparation has been carried out, that the patient is fasting, and perfuse if necessary.

However, the nurse's relationship with the patient is crucial. After ensuring that the necessary equipment is prepared and available to meet all needs and eventualities (scopy, electric scalpel, etc.), the endoscopy nurse ensures that the patient is correctly positioned (on a scopy table or stretcher, in dorsal or lateral decubitus position....).

Endoscopy without general anesthesia is a painful examination for the patient. By providing an appropriate welcome, answering any questions, offering a helping hand and whispering advice on how to cope with the examination, the endoscopy nurse plays an active role in ensuring that the endoscopic procedure is carried out correctly. He or she gives this invasive procedure a touch of humanity, that little air of warmth, contact and accompaniment that turns it from an unpleasant scientific investigation into attentive care.

At the end of the examination, the endoscopy nurse is responsible for monitoring the patient and detecting any complications. The nurse may also play a role in providing psychological support to the patient following the announcement of a painful diagnosis. The nurse may be called upon to answer various questions that still arise after the doctor's explanations, and tries to provide reassurance.

Regarding the general hygiene precautions to be observed by nurses during their participation in digestive endoscopy, several precautions were cited. Cutting fingernails was mentioned by 83% of nurses. Removing watches and jewelry, keeping fingernails short and wearing short-sleeved gowns and masks were cited by 67% of nurses, while over gowns and gloves were cited by 75%, caps by 58% and glasses by 42%.

These data also show a lack of awareness on the part of nurses of the precautions they need to take. Disinfection and hygiene are also an important part of an endoscopy nurse's work.

Numerous regulations govern the disinfection of endoscopes, premises and operating devices. Knowledge and precise application of these texts is essential. In the battle against nosocomial infections waged by medical and health authorities, nurses are the front-line players, helping to prevent contamination, complications and the spread of germs.

On the subject of difficulties, 83% of nurses indicated that they had encountered difficulties influencing the quality of nursing care provided during digestive endoscopy. However, several difficulties were mentioned, including work overload and staff shortages cited by 90% of nurses, equipment shortages cited by 70%, and lack of training cited by 60%.

However, 75% of nurses declare a need for training in equipment maintenance procedures, cited by 82% of them, hygiene precautions mentioned by 58%, and patient preparation for endoscopy mentioned by

RECOMMENDATIONS

Our study revealed a number of misconceptions about the nurse's role in digestive endoscopy.

In view of all these misunderstandings, and to help improve the quality of the nurse's role, we felt it important and beneficial to propose the following recommendations:

- For administration and managers of gastrology departments and digestive endoscopy units or rooms.
    - Supply sufficient equipment for this important practice, specific to the diagnosis and treatment of various digestive pathologies.
    - Ensure good management of human resources and adopt good organization to lighten the load and promote good working conditions.

- For nursing staff
    - Regularly update theoretical and practical knowledge so as to be able to participate safely and appropriately in digestive endoscopy activities.

    - Actively participate in periodically organized continuing education sessions to deepen knowledge and consolidate skills required for patient care in the digestive endoscopy room.

CONCLUSION

Endoscopy is a medical discipline in which the endoscopy nurse plays an important role in patient care before, during and after the examination, in the disinfection and maintenance of medical equipment, and in endoscopic instrumentation. To do so, they must acquire new skills, maintain them through practice, learn about and comply with the various regulations governing the activity, and adapt to a constantly evolving professional field.

Nevertheless, the study we carried out among a sample of nurses working in various gastrology departments revealed a significant lack of knowledge about the various technical and relational activities that nurses must perform in digestive endoscopy rooms.

To remedy this lack of knowledge and improve the quality of the services provided, endoscopy nurses must regularly acquire new knowledge and skills, in addition to the knowledge they have acquired during their training in nursing institutes, to enable them to exercise their role appropriately, actively and safely for their own health and the health of their patients.

BIBLIOGRAPHY

1. ENDOSCOPY, FIBROSCOPY AND COLONOSCOPY. VIDAL 2023.
   https://www.vidal.fr/sante/examens-tests-analyses-medicales/endoscopie-fibroscopie-coloscopie.html

2. From, oesophago-duodenal pathology. "diagnostic indication for upper gastrointestinal endoscopy in adult oesophago-duodenal pathology excluding echo-endoscopy and enteroscopy." (2001).https://www.has-sante.fr/upload/docs/application/pdf/endoscopdigrecos.pdf

3. LEVECQ, Romain. "Comparative cumulative doses of Propofol® during colonoscopies at Poitiers University Hospital following two modes of administration." (2022).https://www.chu-poitiers.fr/specialites/formation-infirmier-anesthesiste/wp-content/uploads/sites/49/2023/03/2022_LEVECQ-Romain.pdf

4. Systchenko, R., Denis Sautereau, and J. M. Canard. "Recommendations of the French Society of Digestive Endoscopy for the organization and operation of a digestive endoscopy technical platform." *ActaEndoscopica* 43 (2013): 198-203. https://www.sfed.org/sites/www.sfed.org/files/2021-10/Plateautechnique_orgafnnt_0.pdf

5. M.BELKAHLA. Diagnostic digestive endoscopy. facmed-univ-oran.dz. https://facmed-univ-oran.dz/ressources/fichiers_produits/fichier_produit_3022.pdf

6. Direction des communications, Ministère de la Santé et des Services sociaux. Endoscopy Unit. https://publications.msss.gouv.qc.ca/msss/fichiers/2015/15-610-03W.pdf

ANNEX

QUESTIONNAIRE

We are .... students of 3ème year nursing at the Université Centrale.
We would like to ask you to answer this questionnaire, which we have designed as part of our
end-of-study project (PFE) entitled :

"THE NURSE'S ROLE IN THE DIGESTIVE ENDOSCOPY ROOM.

The purpose of this questionnaire is purely formative and we guarantee your anonymity.
Thank you very much for your participation, which will certainly be of great interest for the
realization of this end-of-study project.

1. **Genre :**

☐ Men

☐ Woman

2. **Age :**

☐ 20 to 30 years

☐ 31 to 40 years

☐ 41 to 50 years

☐ 51 to 60 years

☐ Over 60

3. **Grade**

☐ Nurse

☐ Senior nurse

☐ Nurse major

☐ Senior nurse major

4. **Seniority in the nursing profession**

☐ Less than 2 years

☐ 2 to 5 years

☐ Over 5 years

5. **Length of service in current department**

☐ Less than 2 years

☐ 2 to 5 years

☐ Over 5 years

6. Have you received specific training in digestive endoscopy?

☐ Yes

☐ No

7. If yes, please specify. What type of training is involved?

☐ Basic training

☐ Continuing education

8. What is digestive endoscopy?

....

....

....

....

9. What are the different types of digestive endoscopy?

....

....

....

....

10. What are the main indications for upper GI endoscopy?

☐ Diagnosis and follow-up of peptic ulcers

☐ Cancer diagnosis and monitoring,

☐ Diagnosis and follow-up of esophageal lesions

☐ Diagnosis and monitoring of gastroesophageal reflux disease,

☐ Diagnosis and follow-up of dysphagia

☐ Diagnosis and follow-up of digestive hemorrhage.

☐ Other: ....

11. What are the main indications for lower GI endoscopy?

☐ Low digestive bleeding (rectorrhagia, melena),

☐ Screening for risk factors for benign colonic tumors (polyps, adenomas)

☐ Risk factor screening for malignant colon tumors (colon cancer)

☐ Screening for inflammatory bowel diseases (Crohn's disease, ulcerative colitis).

☐ Other: ....

12. What are the main risks involved in digestive endoscopy?

☐ Digestive haemorrhage,

☐ Perforation of the digestive wall.

☐ Infection

☐ Respiratory disorders

☐ Cardiovascular disorders

☐ Other: ....

13. What activities do you perform in the digestive endoscopy room?

☐ Assess a clinical situation to organize care management for digestive endoscopy;

☐ Check the functionality of the endoscopic digestive tract;

☐ Participate in the organization and coordination of care activities in complete safety and coherence with the work program;

☐ Provide instrumentation for digestive endoscopy, anticipating needs and being alert to potential risks during the procedure;

☐ Disinfect heat-sensitive materials and evaluate procedures;

☐ Ensure the operational readiness of the endoscope fleet and efficiently manage medical devices;

☐ Participate in analyzing the quality of care and improving professional practices in the digestive endoscopy room;

☐ Other: ....

14. What nursing procedures do you perform before a digestive endoscopy?

☐ Patient reception

☐ Patient set-up

☐ Installation of endoscopic equipment and verification of correct operation

☐ Other: ....

15. What nursing procedures do you perform during a digestive endoscopy?

☐ Assisting the doctor

☐ Connect wall suction.

☐ Monitor scope and patient,

☐ Inform the doctor of any incident

☐ Other: ....

16. What nursing procedures do you perform after a digestive endoscopy?

☐ Reinstall the patient.

☐ Arranging equipment

☐ Dispose of contaminated materials.

☐ Wash your hands.

☐ Ensuring traceability of care

☐ Other: ....

17. What are the general hygiene precautions you should observe when taking part in a digestive endoscopy?

☐ Short sleeve

☐ No watches or jewelry on hands

☐ Short-cut nails

☐ Wearing gloves

☐ Wearing glasses

☐ Wearing a mask

☐ Port de charlotte

☐ Wearing overblouses

☐ Other: ....

18. Do you ensure endoscope disinfection in your digestive endoscopy room?

☐ Yes

☐ No

19. If yes. What endoscope disinfection procedures do you use in your digestive endoscopy room?

20. If you use strictly manual disinfection. What are the steps in this disinfection procedure?

....

....

....

....

....

21. If you use assisted manual disinfection. What are the steps in this disinfection procedure?

....

....

....

....

....

22. If you use automated disinfection. What are the steps in this disinfection procedure?

....

....

....

....

....

23. Have you encountered any difficulties that affect the quality of nursing care provided during a digestive endoscopy?

☐ Yes

☐ No

24. If so, what are these difficulties?

☐ Lack of training

☐ Work overload

☐ Lack of personnel

☐ Lack of equipment

☐ Other: ....

25. Do you need additional training in digestive endoscopy?

☐ Yes

☐ No

26. If so, what topics would you like to be trained in?

....

....

....

....

....

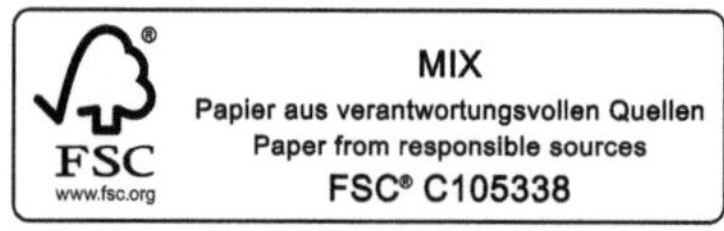

Printed by Books on Demand GmbH, Norderstedt / Germany